Everything Apple Cider Vinegar

Any and Everything about Apple Cider Vinegar

Apple Cider Vinegar is the best thing poppin right now. It is for a variety of uses. There is so much to know about Apple Cider Vinegar. In this book, you will be intrigued and compelled to keep on reading. Wait until you see what all the fuss is about.

Are Apple Cider Vinegar Gummies Legit for Weight Loss?

You might think you've seen it all when it comes to apple cider vinegar. And that's fair enough, considering it appears on Instagram in everything from simple salad dressings to influencers' "fat-burning" elixirs. But these days, the substance is taking yet another form: apple cider vinegar *gummies*.

Think of it as your daily multi-gummy reimagined to deliver the supposed benefits of apple cider vinegar. They tend to have around 500 milligrams (equivalent to a few teaspoons) of ACV per serving, but other ingredients vary from brand to brand. BeLive, for instance, boasts a sugar-free recipe, and Goli claims its formula includes vitamins B9 and B12.

The appeal is clear: The gummies are, in theory, a more pleasant way to incorporate apple cider vinegar into your diet than, say, drinking the stuff raw or swallowing the supp in pill form. In fact, the great taste of Goli gummies comes up in a ton of Amazon reviews, along with other words of praise. Users claim they have plenty of benefits, from reducing bloat to curbing appetite. But are they really all they're cracked up to be?

What do apple cider vinegar gummies supposedly do?

Before we dive in, keep in mind that there's an important distinction between apple cider vinegar in its raw, unfiltered form and tacky form. "We don't necessarily know that the gummies are doing anything, because there's no research on them," Meshulam says. Bottom line: Any health benefits associated with apple cider vinegar haven't been linked to the actual gummy kind yet.

Here's what we know about the main claims attached to apple cider vinegar in liquid or oral supplement form.

Help you lose weight

Apple cider vinegar on its own isn't going to be a magic pill for weight loss, but it *might* give you an edge if you're already working towards a weight-loss goal via nutrition and exercise changes. There's some interesting research out there on this front, but it comes with a few caveats. More on that later.

Strengthen your gut health

You might see claims that apple cider vinegar has prebiotic or probiotic properties. Quick refresher: Probiotics are the "good" bacteria in your gut that support digestive health and your immune system. Meanwhile, prebiotics "feed" those bacteria.

The ACV fermentation process does create bacteria, However, for something to be considered a probiotic, it must have enough healthy bacteria to promote a health benefit. *And while apples are rich in pectin, a prebiotic, a tablespoon of apple cider vinegar (two gummies, depending on the brand) does not have enough of the fiber to count as your dose of prebiotics for the day.* Put simply, do not rely on ACV alone to support the healthy bacteria in your gut.

Still, it can aid digestion: The acetic acid in apple cider vinegar can help people with low levels of stomach acid to break down food. Plus, ACV can promote motility, —in other words, it keeps things moving in your GI system.

Support your immune system
Probiotics (and the prebiotics supporting them) *are* good for your immune system. The good bacteria can basically "nudge out" harmful bacteria, and some probiotics boost the production of antibodies. But again, don't rely on ACV alone to support these beneficial bacteria.

Support heart health
Acetic acid helped to lower "bad" cholesterol in rats while raising their "good" cholesterol in one older study. The study didn't include people, though, so take the results with a grain of salt.

Boost your energy
Apple cider vinegar doesn't have a special nutrient that should make you feel more energetic. However, ACV could provide more *consistent* energy throughout the day by preventing blood sugar spikes (and the crashes that come along with them, which make you feel exhausted), she explains.

Side note: Some brands (like Goli, Garden of Life, and Vitafusion) say their ACV gummies include as much as 250 percent of your daily rec for vitamin B12. Since a B12 deficiency can cause tiredness, they could help your energy level if you're deficient. But this is probably not the case if you're someone who eats animal-based products.

Improve your skin
ACV has anti-inflammatory properties, and your skin can reap the benefits, given that skin issues like acne and redness are signs of inflammation. Still, it's not the first thing you should turn to if you're hoping to boost your skin health.

Relieve heartburn
ACV might help with heartburn (since the moderate acid could, in theory, bring down the pH of your stomach). But the study at the heart of this claim wasn't peer-reviewed or published. There's no data in medical journals indicating that apple cider vinegar can safely or effectively relieve heartburn, according to Harvard Medical School, and most evidence is anecdotal, so the effectiveness will depend on the person.

Reduce bloating
It's not always clear what's causing bloat, but one potential culprit is small intestinal bacterial overgrowth (which can result in "bad" bacteria creating gas), according to Harvard Medical School. ACV "creates an environment where good bacteria is more fruitful," and the good bacteria kills bad bacteria.

Detoxify the body
This is one of those claims that *isn't* supported by science in any way. "The truth is, if you have a healthy, working liver and healthy, working kidneys, your body is naturally detoxifying all day, every day on its own. You don't need a supplement to do that for you.

You might also see claims that ACV can clean out your arteries, but let's be clear: This isn't legit. The idea, according to Harvard Medical School, is that a substance related to acetic acid can pull metals out of the bloodstream, so ingesting ACV could help dissolve plaque in the arteries. But as Harvard Medical School explains, don't buy into these unproven claims.

Do apple cider vinegar gummies help with weight loss?
There is some research linking apple cider vinegar consumption and weight loss, but the relevant studies tend to be small. One, for instance, published by the *Journal of Functional Foods* in 2018, took place over 12 weeks (about 3 months) and included 39 participants. All the subjects followed a restricted calorie diet, but some of them also consumed apple cider vinegar—and they lost more weight.

There are a couple of ways through which ACV could help you shed pounds. For one thing, the acetic acid may help keep food in your stomach for longer, and therefore keep you feeling satiated. Blood sugar regulation also comes back into play here. When our blood sugar spikes high, insulin is released to lower it. And insulin is also a hormone that tells your body there's a ton of food available. So, in theory, if blood sugar isn't spiking all the time, this fat storage hormone isn't being released as much either.

Ultimately, there's good news and bad news when it comes to weight loss and the ACV *gummies*. On the plus side, they should contain enough apple cider vinegar to be beneficial per relevant research findings. For instance, some studies had people consuming two tablespoons of ACV per day—that's about four Goli gummies, and you can take up to six. But appetite suppression may be somewhat related to the vinegar taste, and you won't get that with a sweet gummy.

Again, there's no magic pill (or in this case, gummy). Incorporating ACV into an otherwise unhealthy diet won't lead to weight loss—what you're eating matters.

Are there side effects of taking ACV gummies?
One thing to note is that gummies have added ingredients. "The gummies usually come with a good amount of sugar, and a lot of other stabilizers and things to get it in that gummy form. These things aren't always harmful or even bad, but her thought is that it's best to keep nutrition as simple as possible. Plus, supplements aren't regulated by the FDA, so we don't really know everything that might be in them.

As for ACV in general, it can interact with some supplements and drugs, like diuretics and insulin, according to the Mayo Clinic. People with diabetes should avoid taking ACV products like this, as they can lower your blood sugar, and pregnant and breastfeeding women should also skip them.

Bottom line: Make sure to talk to your doctor before starting to take any new supplement.

So, should I buy apple cider vinegar gummies?
You may be better off saving your money. It's better to buy a bottle of the actual vinegar if you want to incorporate ACV into your diet. "I would always, always, always opt for the actual food version, because you know what's in it.

But don't take a shot of raw apple cider vinegar, as it can hurt your esophagus. Instead, try putting a few teaspoons in your salad dressing, marinades, or sparkling water if you're interested in incorporating ACV into a nutritious diet.

Apple Cider Vinegar Pills: Are There Health Benefits?

Apple cider vinegar is made from fermented apple juice. It has a wide range of culinary applications, from salad dressings to marinades, and is also a popular folk remedy for a variety of conditions. In 1958, a physician named D.C. Jarvis recommended a health tonic made from apple cider vinegar and honey.

Recently, apple cider vinegar has been touted as a weight loss tonic, as a remedy for acid reflux, and even as a hair rinse. While modern science has lent some support to these and other claims about apple cider vinegar, much more research is needed to determine whether apple cider vinegar pills are a beneficial part of a daily regimen.

Nutrition Information
One tablespoon of unfiltered apple cider vinegar contains:

- Calories: 7
- Protein: 0 grams
- Fat: 0 grams
- Carbohydrates: 2 grams
- Fiber: 0 grams
- Sugar: 0 grams

Apple cider vinegar is not a significant source of other nutrients.

Potential Health Benefits of Apple Cider Vinegar Pills
Research has found a few potential health benefits from taking apple cider vinegar pills:

Antimicrobial Effects

Apple cider vinegar is used in a variety of folk remedies as an antibacterial and antifungal agent, and scientific research supports these claims. One study found strong antibacterial activity in apple cider concentrations of 25 percent.

Another found significant therapeutic implications for treatment of E. coli, staph infections, and yeast infections.

Apple cider vinegar has even been shown to treat vaginal yeast infections that did not respond to other forms of medical treatment.

Diabetes Management

Apple cider vinegar pills may help improve glycemic control (effect on blood sugar) in patients with diabetes since they have been shown to have an anti-glycemic effect.

Especially when taken at mealtimes, apple cider vinegar can also reduce fasting blood glucose concentrations in healthy adults at risk for type II diabetes.

For people with diabetes, apple cider vinegar can also help improve hemoglobin A1C values (blood sugar attached to red blood cells) when taken regularly.

Metabolism and Weight Loss

There is some evidence to show that taking apple cider vinegar pills can improve glucose metabolism, lipid profiles, and body weight overall.

Much more research is needed to prove a conclusive effect of apple cider vinegar on metabolism and weight loss, but several studies have indicated that it has a beneficial effect.

Potential Risks of Apple Cider Vinegar Pills
You should consult with your doctor before taking apple cider vinegar pills or any other supplement. Consider the following before adding apple cider vinegar pills to your regimen:

Nausea

Ingestion of vinegar, including apple cider vinegar, may stimulate nausea in people with sensitive stomachs. If you experience nausea as a result of taking apple cider vinegars, speak to your doctor about finding an alternative.

Pregnancy Concerns

The effects of apple cider vinegar pills on someone who is pregnant, or breast-feeding are inconclusive. If you're pregnant or breastfeeding a baby, it is best to look for an alternative.

Medication Interference

Avoid apple cider vinegar pills if you're already taking a diuretic as their actions may be compounded. Since apple cider vinegar has natural diuretic properties, it may interfere with the action of lithium and similar medications.

Apple cider vinegar pills should also be avoided if you're taking other medications that reduce potassium in the body, like Digoxin and Insulin.

11 Side Effects of Apple Cider Vinegar When Used in Excess

ACV is being recommended by dietitians and health-conscious people who consider it as an all-in-one natural cure for several diseases ranging from weight loss to ulcers. Apple cider vinegar translates to 'sour wine of apple' in some languages. This sour juice is packed full of essential vitamins and minerals like pectin, folic acid, biotin, pantothenic acid, vitamins B1, B2, B6, and C, niacin, sodium, phosphorus, iron, calcium, potassium, magnesium, and acetic acid.

Side Effects of Apple Cider Vinegar

In most studies, the side effects of ACV have been caused by excess dosages. It is important that the prescribed amount is always taken. It is very important that a healthcare provider should be consulted before taking Apple Cider Vinegar.

How Much Apple Cider Vinegar Is Safe to Consume?

The recommended dose of ACV varies depending on the individual needs. If you want to take advantage of the actual health benefits of ACV, mix two tablespoons of ACV with a cup of water and consume it once a day. Experts recommend consuming ACV with a straw to avoid it coming in contact with your teeth.

Let us look at the side effects caused by excess consumption of apple cider vinegar.

1. Low Blood Sugar Levels

The excessive use of ACV can lower the blood sugar levels as it counteracts the accumulation of excess sugar in the blood. It may cause diabetic hypoglycemia, cutting off glucose supply to the brain, and resulting in unconsciousness and even coma, in some cases. However, people suffering from type II diabetes and insulin resistance might find this activity of apple cider vinegar as a blessing.

2. Acne

One of the many purposes of taking ACV is to flush out toxins from the system. However, it can lead to acne production since the body tends to expel toxins via our skin.

3. Headaches and Nausea

The excessive use of ACV can lead to painful headaches accompanied by a feeling of nausea. This occurs because of its detoxification property that makes the brain release harmful toxins. Make sure to dilute this product before consuming it.

4. Reactions to Certain Medications

Since it is acidic in nature, ACV can easily react negatively with certain drugs like diuretics, laxatives, and insulin. It has a direct effect on insulin levels and blood sugar. Any person suffering from any health disorder should consult with their doctor before consuming ACV, as it may prove to be highly hazardous when taken with blood pressure and diabetes medications.

5. Stomach Problems

If you are using ACV for detoxification, it might cause serious diarrhea, indigestion, and heartburn due to the acidic nature of ACV. It is advised to lower the dosage if these side effects do not subside naturally.

6. Tooth Enamel Damage

Consuming undiluted ACV orally can destroy your tooth enamel, because of the high acidic level it contains, giving it a yellowish tinge. Additionally, it increases your dental sensitivity as well. Consume liquid diluted ACV using a straw and brush your teeth immediately after intake.

7. Decreased Bone Density

The excessive use of apple cider vinegar might reduce the bone mineral density, causing your bones to be weak and brittle. People suffering from osteoporosis should consult a physician before consuming ACV.

8. A Sore Throat

The oral overuse of apple cider vinegar can eventually lead to throat irritation, caused mainly due to the presence of acetic acid in apple cider vinegar. Always dilute apple cider vinegar in water, if you are planning to use it for a prolonged period. It helps prevent the damage to our esophageal wall.

9. Tissue Damage

The excessive use of ACV may cause damage to the esophagus, tooth enamel, and stomach lining due to the high level of citric acidic content in it. Moreover, direct application of undiluted apple cider vinegar on the skin can cause irritation, rashes, and a burning sensation. It is very important to always dilute before use.

10. Decreased Potassium Levels

The high acetic acid content of ACV causes low potassium levels in the blood. This condition is called hypokalemia and may cause many associated symptoms and ailments including nausea, cramps, weakness, frequent urination, low blood pressure, changes in heart rhythm, and paralysis.

11. Lowered Mineral Levels

Using ACV to detoxify, flushes out both good and bad substances from the body. It expels a few essential nutrients like minerals which are very important for health. Prevent this from happening by taking a daily dose of multivitamins.

Consuming ACV in the correct dosages may prevent and avoid all the above-mentioned side effects.

Results will differ for everyone, depending on existing health factors, lifestyle and physical condition. The information contained on this site is for informational purposes only and is not a substitute for medical advice provided by your doctor or physician. The information, we provide should not be used for diagnosis, treatment or prevention of any disease. Testimonials and results contained are reflective of the typical examples consumers experienced and may not be an implication of future results for you. These statements have not been evaluated by the Food and Drug Administration.

Top Tips When Taking Apple Cider Vinegar

As this wonder drink has gained a lot of popularity in recent years, Apple Cider Vinegar, (ACV) has become very popular and is being recommended by dietitians and health-conscious people who consider it as an all-in-one natural cure for several diseases. Drinking ACV aids weight loss keeps blood sugar in check, boosts health and helps in improving acne and scars. Despite all the numerous benefits, health experts warn us to practice caution. It should never be taken in excess, should be diluted for oral and topical use and never be taken undiluted.

How Much Is the Recommended Dosage?
The recommended dose of ACV varies depending on what the individual's needs are. The actual health benefits dosage recommendation is to mix two tablespoons of ACV in a glass of water and consume it once a day.

1. Drink ACV Undiluted
Consuming undiluted ACV may produce a vast amount of health issues. Consuming undiluted ACV orally can destroy your tooth enamel, because of the high acidic level it contains, giving it a yellowish tinge. Additionally, it increases your dental sensitivity as well. Consume liquid diluted ACV using a straw and brush your teeth immediately after intake.

2. Drink Too Much
Drinking too much ACV may lead to many health problems which prove to be dangerous to the body. These health problems are:

- Low Blood Sugar Levels
- Headaches & Nausea
- Gastrointestinal Problems
- Decreased Bone Density
- A Sore Throat
- Tissue Damage
- Low Potassium Levels
- Decreased Mineral Levels

As its numerous benefits are known, so are their health issues which may occur if too much ACV is consumed. It is crucial that not go beyond two tablespoons a day – diluted in water, drink of choice or a smoothie.

3. Drink It Right After Eating Food
Taking ACV directly after eating food is not healthy as it may delay your digestion process. It is advisable to wait for at least 20 to 25 minutes before taking it. ACV improves digestion by

keeping food in the stomach for longer, which allows more time for the stomach acid to do its job before sending the remains into the small intestines. Drinking ACV on an empty stomach maximizes health benefits and boosts the ability to process food.

4. Inhale ACV

Avoid inhaling ACV as it might cause damage to your lungs. Rather avoid inhaling it as it could cause burning sensation in your lungs.

5. Drink It Right Before Bedtime

Consuming ACV before sleeping is not a good idea. Health experts say that drinking apple cider vinegar before bed can harm the esophagus. And as an additional bonus, your bladder might keep u up all night.

6. Apply It Undiluted on The Skin

ACV is indeed a natural treatment for blemishes and infections of the skin, but just as it may burn the throat, it may also cause a slight burning sensation in the skin. People with sensitive skin or with any skin condition should take special care before applying ACV topically. It should always be diluted.

7. Take ACV If You Have Helicobacter Pylori

ACV can, for the most part, seriously boost your digestive health. But it has been proven that there are some stomach conditions that this acidic substance will only make worse. For instance, if you have Helicobacter pylori (the bacteria linked to peptic ulcers) ACV should be avoided as it may cause even more irritation.

8. Take ACV Without Consulting with Your Doctor

If you are considering taking ACV and you have a medical condition or are on any kind of medication, it is advised to consult with your doctor and seek professional advice before consuming this product.

Apple Cider Vinegar Side Effects
Are There Any Effects Users Should Be Aware Of?
Apple cider vinegar (ACV) is extremely beneficial and is used as a main staple in many folk remedies around the world. However, that doesn't mean you won't experience any unnatural effects upon ingestion. As everyone differs, we have found that ACV does not have an agreeable effect on some people's stomach. What then could the side effects of ACV be? Should you, the user, be concerned?

The acetic acid in ACV is the main cause of side effects, and that is what some people are sensitive to. ACV also contains prebiotics, which may have a few minor effects as well. More detail on this is given below.

Possible Apple Cider Vinegar Side Effects
We would like to point out that any unpleasant experiences typically only occur in large doses or an overdose. Unless your stomach is especially sensitive or you have had a medical condition, you should be fine if you stick to recommended servings.

Throat Burn
ACV should always be diluted and never be taken in its pure natural form, especially if you are sensitive to acidic foods. Acetic acid is acidic, and some people, and children have experienced a mild but noticeable burning sensation in their throat.

Teeth Erosion/Sensitive Teeth
Acidic and citric foods may have an effect on your oral health, which might strip away teeth enamel causing sensitive teeth. After consuming acidic foods, drink some water or rinse the mouth with water to dilute the acid. You can also chew sugarless gum; the chewing stimulates saliva flow which in turn reduces the acid.

Skin Burns
Some people use ACV topically to treat or remove skin blemishes, such as acne.
ACV side effects also include skin burns if applied topically. ACV is indeed a natural treatment for skin blemishes, but just as it may burn the throat, it may also cause a slight burning sensation on the skin. People with sensitive skin or with any skin condition should take special care before applying ACV topically.

Nausea
The vinegar in ACV may cause nausea. In certain cases, some people who consumed the vinegar reported feeling nauseous accompanied by a loss of appetite. It's believed that nausea and subsequent appetite loss were due to the sour, sharp, unpleasant taste of the vinegar. People sensitive to the taste of vinegar may experience small degrees of nausea and hunger loss.

Digestion Problems in People with Type 1 Diabetes
ACV is celebrated for reducing digestion problems and alleviating irritable bowel syndrome. However, in very rare instances, it may induce the opposite for people with type I diabetes. ACV improves digestion by keeping food in the stomach for longer, which allows more time for the stomach acid to do its job before sending the remains into the small intestines.

However, in the case of diabetics, this may worsen pre-existing symptoms of gastroparesis. It is a condition that hinders the function of nerves in the stomach and intestinal lining. Which causes food to remain in the stomach longer than it should, and it leads to symptoms of bloating and heartburn.

Abdominal Pain

ACV contains prebiotics, which is a very good thing since prebiotics are necessary for probiotic health. However, a small minority of people have reported prebiotics side effects, such as abdominal pain, bloating and gas. Certain prebiotics may enlarge the number of gas-producing bacteria, hence the bloating. There is no reason why you should experience severe prebiotics side effects, as long as you are healthy and only consume the recommended dosages.

Should You Be Concerned?

People who experienced undesirable effects usually either consumed high doses of ACV or had pre-existing medical conditions. Even if you experience unpleasant sensations in the beginning, they will most likely disappear once your body adjusts. Ultimately, the scientific health benefits far outweigh potential side effects. I believe you'll be amazed at how much better you feel after making ACV a regular part of your dietary regimen. ACV may be obtained in liquid form or in tablet form.

Why Should You Drink Apple Cider Vinegar in the Morning?

Apple cider vinegar, known as ACV, is the latest in a long list of health trends. The best kind being with Mother which means you are getting unrefined, unpasteurized and unfiltered ACV. The "Mother" is a colony of beneficial bacteria which helps to maintain a healthy alkaline pH level, eases digestive ailments, accelerates weight loss, helps to regulate blood sugar, can help lower blood pressure, improves heart health, promotes healthy detoxification of the liver and other organs, eliminates candida overgrowth, can help prevent osteoporosis, slows the aging process, provides a glowing skin, assists in the fight against free radical damage, to name but a few benefits.

How to Drink Apple Cider Vinegar

Drinking apple cider vinegar first thing in the morning is the best way to take advantage of its many health benefits, but it can be difficult to do, especially when it is the first thing you are consuming. It might take some getting used to initially, but once you get used to the taste, it is hard to go without it.

There are many ways to drink apple cider vinegar in the morning to make it easier, you don't have to drink it straight. You can incorporate it with other fruit juices, as a smoothie or as a hot drink. Mix one teaspoon with a cup of warm water and a little honey if necessary, to taste, then stir the drink and allow it to steep for a few minutes before drinking. After steeping, drink it slowly like a cup of tea. ACV should be taken at least a half an hour before eating breakfast.

Ways to Incorporate ACV into Drinks

ACV can be mixed with honey

Mix it with horseradish and Habanero peppers – Fiery one!

Try it with crushed strawberries and mint

Mix with maple syrup, ground ginger, and water

Mix with crushed berries and lemon with a dollop of honey

Mix with watermelon and honey

Mix with blueberries, strawberries, banana, and water – as a smoothie

Additional Health Benefits

Combining ACV with certain spices, herbs, and fruits provide even more additional health benefits, such as:

Watermelon and basil – For a detox

Turmeric (fights inflammation) tea with honey – For a detox

Aloe vera, kiwi and cucumbers – For healthy skin and nails

Grape with Seltzer water and kombucha – For anti-aging and gut health

Chamomile tea – For reducing stress

Strawberry and lemon – For increased energy

Pear, raspberries, blackberries and purified water (full of vitamins A, C, and K, iron, magnesium, and phosphorus) – For aiding digestion

Is Timing Important?

First thing in the morning is the best time to drink apple cider vinegar. Some of the key benefits to drinking it in the morning are that it boosts metabolism and weight loss, and it helps with sugar cravings throughout the day (controls appetite), as well as controls cholesterol and treats unsightly blemishes, itchy insect bites and sunburns, and promotes healthy skin, hair, and nails. However, you can choose to drink it whenever you like.

If you prefer to drink it before bed, you may find that you may need to use the bathroom a lot through the night. There are some mixes and a handful of teas you could drink at night for certain ailments (such as aches and pains, from muscle soreness to chronic headaches). If needed, ACV may be taken at night to help ease certain ailments.

Can ACV Help Digestion?
Apple cider vinegar is becoming well known for its weight-loss benefits and fat reducing properties. The mere fact alone that it reduces fat deposits in the body makes it great for

detoxification because it reduces the risk of developing cardiovascular disease. But there are other detox benefits of apple cider vinegar too.

Apple cider vinegar is a great addition to any detox program because it is rich in antioxidants, nutrients, and enzymes but it's important to use organic apple cider vinegar that still has "the mother" in it. The mother refers to leftover pulp from the apples that made the vinegar.

It clears the digestive system

Because it is acidic and that it has natural probiotic abilities, apple cider vinegar is great for clearing out the intestine and helping it to function better. All these things help to reduce both constipation and diarrhea as well as indigestion. Clearing out the intestine is important in any detox program because many of the toxins are going to be excreted that way. Clearing the digestive tract also makes way for other detox compounds and normal nutrients to be absorbed.

It's a source of natural enzymes

An enzyme is basically a protein that is very chemically reactive and helps to break large biomolecules down (or build them up)? Enzymes are very useful in digesting food. The enzymes in apple cider vinegar don't directly help to break down food, but they do promote the growth of good bacteria in the intestine and these bacteria improve digestion through the release of their own enzymes. This also helps to reduce the number of harmful bacteria, which in turn reduces the risk of gastrointestinal problems.

It's also a source of vitamins and minerals

Apple cider vinegar is full of different kinds of vitamins and minerals. Vitamins and minerals are important for all parts of the detox process, but they mainly assist the bodies enzymes to do their job. Some toxins are unable to be excreted until they are broken down by some of the body's enzymes in the liver. Vitamins and minerals are also important for the immune system to fight off bacterial and viral toxins. It is also possible that during the detox process, you are flushing out some of the good nutrients – and apple cider vinegar will replace those.

It reduces mucus

Mucus builds up in the sinuses can be a sign of toxin build up. This is because the body naturally produces mucus to form a protective layer against contaminants. When mucus-secreting cells are under a lot of stress, mucus secretion can become too much and cause more harm than benefit.

Apple cider vinegar helps to break up this mucus so that the body can eliminate it. An overflow of mucus can also just leave you feeling down and unwell. It affects your breathing and gives you headaches. Apple cider vinegar, therefore, helps to get rid of these symptoms by breaking up the mucus.

The Powerful Combination of Turmeric and Apple Cider Vinegar

Both apple cider vinegar and turmeric are known for the variety of health benefits they provide. But what happens when you mix the two superfoods together? The benefits would be amazing. He developed a recipe that combines turmeric and apple cider vinegar as one healthy daily tonic.

I believe the combination is excellent for the bacteria in the intestine and for reducing inflammation in the body. Their individual benefits combined to create one of the most potent anti-inflammatory health foods that are completely natural as well.

Benefits of apple cider vinegar

Apple cider vinegar has been used for centuries in natural medicine and as part of the diet. But recently there have been some scientifically proven benefits derived from taking apple cider vinegar every day.

A group of studies has determined that daily apple cider vinegar is able to assist with weight loss. Apple cider vinegar is directly able to reduce the storage of fat in the body and so cause a reduction in total body fat.

It also helps to reduce blood glucose levels and blood cholesterol levels. These reductions significantly lower the risk of developing cardiovascular diseases, diabetes and even cancer.

Benefits of turmeric

Turmeric is one of the most anti-inflammatory herbs that exist. Turmeric directly inhibits one of the enzymes responsible for the main inflammatory pathway in the body. Similarly, to aspirin, it reduces the effect of an enzyme called COX-2. COX-2 is mostly responsible for creating pain and inflammation, so inhibiting it helps to reduce inflammation in the body, which also reduces the risk of developing inflammatory diseases like cardiovascular disease.

The pigment in turmeric, called curcumin is also a powerful antioxidant. Antioxidants reduce inflammation in a different way. They react with environmental and body toxins that are normally responsible for destroying cell membranes. When these toxins react with antioxidants instead, they don't cause any damage to the cells.

Synergistic effects

The belief is that turmeric and apple cider vinegar combine in what's called a synergistic effect. When two compounds are mixed, they can either negatively affect each other or positively affect each other. In this case, turmeric and apple cider vinegar positively affect each other. When compounds positively affect each other, they can either have an additive effect, where their effects add up to produce double effectiveness, or as in this case, they can be synergistic, where their combined effects are even more than double effective. It makes sense too when you think about the different ways, they work to reduce inflammation and the risk of chronic diseases.

The turmeric and apple cider vinegar shot

To make the tonic you need:

⅖ cup (3.4 fl oz) of any fruit juice

1 tablespoon ground turmeric

½ teaspoon ground black pepper

1 teaspoon ground cinnamon

1 pinch ground cloves

1 tablespoon apple cider vinegar

1 tablespoon olive oil

1 tablespoon freshly squeezed lemon juice

Stir all the ingredients together and drink the mixture as quickly as possible following with a glass of water. This concoction can be taken once or twice a day, in the morning and/or in the evening.

Why You Should Try an Apple Cider Vinegar Cleanse

The apple cider vinegar cleanse has taken the internet by storm as several celebrities and high-profile doctors swear by its health benefits. Apple cider vinegar has been used in natural medicine and nutrition for many decades now and there are several claims that it supports the health in a variety of ways.

It's called the apple cider cleanse because it helps the body to get rid of some of the most unwanted molecules like fats and cholesterol. Many experts are opposed to classifying apple cider vinegar as a "cure-all", but they do agree on certain health benefits that apple cider vinegar provides based on scientific research.

Weight loss

Weight loss studies have been conducted in both animals and humans and the definitive result is that apple cider vinegar can help a person lose weight. Scientists believe, based on the animal studies, that the acetic acid in apple cider vinegar inhibits certain enzymes that are responsible for storing fat. There is also the study that shows how apple cider vinegar slows the movement of food through the digestive tract which could, in theory, help a person feel fuller for longer. The weight loss isn't major, so it can't reverse bad eating habits, but it does give a boost to your diet.

Regulating blood sugar

One of the great proven benefits of apple cider vinegar is that it helps to regulate blood sugar. The amount of sugar in the blood spikes after a person has eaten a meal, especially if it contains a lot of carbohydrates. High levels of sugar in the blood for long periods of time can be damaging to the body because they are stored as fat and they can cause insulin resistance. Recent research has also shown that high blood sugar levels can cause chronic inflammation which increases the risk of heart disease and cancer. Scientists have found that acetic acid, the same component that reduced fat storage, also helps the various cells of the body to take up glucose (sugar), leading to a reduced amount of it in the blood.

It's good for the heart

Apart from reducing blood sugar, apple cider vinegar has also been shown to be protective of the heart by reducing cholesterol. Cholesterol is a type of fat that deposits into the walls of blood vessels and makes them stiff. This is a major risk factor for a heart attack, and it can also increase your blood pressure. Since apple cider vinegar helps to break down fats, it also helps to break down cholesterol and protect the heart and may have an indirect effect on blood pressure.

Apple cider vinegar tonic

The traditional apple cider vinegar tonic consists of 2 teaspoons of apple cider vinegar diluted in 8 oz of water. Many people add honey or cinnamon and some even cayenne pepper to change up the taste a little bit. Some of these natural flavorings may also provide their own health benefits. It is important to drink the apple cider vinegar in a diluted form and not pure because otherwise it can cause harm.

The Different Ways to Take Apple Cider Vinegar

There are many claims about how apple cider vinegar can help with your general health. The key is all the enzymes, vitamins and minerals locked up in the unrefined pulp. All these great nutrients are perfect for detoxing and can assist with weight loss, reducing blood sugar, reducing circulating cholesterol and fat and enhancing the immune system.

The following recipes contain 1 to 2 teaspoons of apple cider vinegar, the right dosage needed to achieve all these benefits. Combining apple cider vinegar with other healthy foods like fruit juices and herbs, might even enhance the health benefits and it will taste great too!

The classic

Classically, 1 to 2 spoons of apple cider vinegar are mixed with 8 ounces of water and flavored with different things- like lemon juice, cayenne pepper or honey. It's a very simple and easy solution to make and it is one of the best-known recipes. The cinnamon also helps to reduce fat and improve digestion, and cayenne pepper helps to speed up the metabolism.

Mix it with some juice

Apple cider vinegar also works great when mixed with three quarters of a cup of cranberry juice and three quarters of a cup of water. Cranberry juice is very high in antioxidants, which come with their own set of health benefits like reducing inflammation and slowing down aging. There is some evidence that cranberry juice helps to clear the kidneys of toxins and remove fat from the lymphatic system.

Another good combination is 2 teaspoons of apple cider vinegar in a cup of grapefruit juice with a bit of honey to taste. Grapefruit juice is also rich in antioxidants and it helps to lower blood pressure.

Mixing apple cider vinegar with limeade makes a delicious drink that the whole family will love. This drink has a high sugar content so it should not be consumed as often as other recipes. All it takes to make as 1 cup of water 2 teaspoons of apple cider, vinegar and 6 teaspoons of limeade concentrate.

Have it in a smoothie

There are several different ways to incorporate apple cider vinegar into a smoothie. One option is to blend 1 teaspoon of apple cider vinegar with the quarter cup of water, a whole cup of cut apples and 2 teaspoons of avocado. Throw in a quarter cup of ice to get the right texture.

Some other great health foods to go along with the apple cider vinegar are berries. Try making a berry apple cider vinegar smoothie by mixing a cup of frozen berries, one banana, a cup of almond milk and 2 teaspoons of apple cider vinegar.

Try it with some green tea

Green tea is also hailed as one of a group of superfoods. Green tea is also stuffed with nutrients and antioxidants. Mix 1 cup of green tea with 1 teaspoon of apple cider vinegar and add honey and mint to taste and you've got yourself powerfully healthy combination.

Top Uses of Apple Cider Vinegar

Some people enjoy apple cider vinegar as a dressing for their foods. But recently, people have started exploring apple cider vinegar as a whole lot more than a condiment. There have been claims for several centuries that apple cider vinegar can promote a person's health and well-being and provide a variety of health benefits.

What makes apple cider vinegar quite unique is the fact that certain organic formulations contain the original pulp of the apple, which when fermented, is referred to as "the mother". This part of the apple cider vinegar is rich in vitamins, minerals enzymes, and even probiotic bacteria.

The claimed benefits of apple cider vinegar
All the nutrients in apple cider vinegar have the potential to cause great health benefits for the body. Some of the suggested benefits of apple cider vinegar include:

- Improved potassium intake
- Improved immune system functioning due to vitamins
- Weight loss
- Body pH balance
- Assisting digestion
- Improving the gut microbiome
- Maintaining the health of the skin, including reducing acne
- Reducing appetite
- Assistance with cholesterol
- Controlling diabetes type 2
- Removing "sludge toxins" from the body

Many of these claims are anecdotal and a lot more research is needed but there are a few benefits that are proven by science.

What the science says
There are a few small-scale studies that have researched the effect of apple cider vinegar in relation to some health factors. Participants who took apple cider vinegar significantly lowered their blood glucose. The participants also reported that their appetite was produced after consuming a meal with apple cider vinegar.

There is also a study that proved that apple cider vinegar reduced body weight and total fats in its participants. A reduction in the amount of circulating fats also reduces the risk of atherosclerosis, the hardening of arteries, which in turn reduces the risk of having a heart attack or stroke.

Most of the proven health benefits provided by apple cider vinegar reduce the risk of developing metabolic syndrome, which is essentially an unhealthy state where the body is filled with toxins and is quite pro-inflammatory.

How to detox with apple cider vinegar

One of the recipes for a detox solution is made by mixing one or two tablespoons of unfiltered apple cider vinegar with 8 ounces of water and then adding one or two teaspoons of honey or stevia. Some recipes also contain lemon juice or pepper. Generally, this solution is taken three times a day: when getting out of bed, in the mid-morning and in the midafternoon.

Some considerations

It's important to make sure that the apple cider vinegar is diluted, or it could cause some serious side effects like tooth erosion and burning in the throat. It is also important to consult your doctor if you are taking any medications, as apple cider vinegar could interfere with that. Any sort of long-term health conditions like diabetes or even pregnancy might also be affected differently by the detox, so be sure to consult.

Detox Your Body with ACV

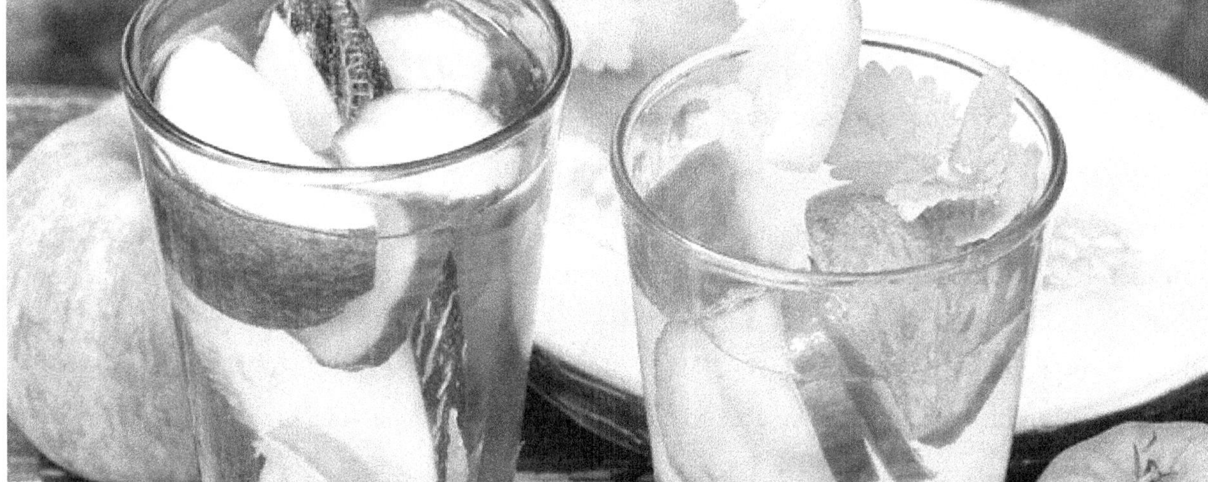

With living our busy lives, it can become tough to keep a nutritious diet, get the recommended number of workouts, and follow a healthy lifestyle in general. Because of this, sometimes our bodies need a little extra help getting rid of excess toxins. But now, there are ways to do this from the comfort of your own home, with things you may already have in your kitchen.

When to Detox?
Sometimes it is difficult to know when our bodies need extra help, especially with detoxifying. There are simple tips to take notice of, which could be your body's way of asking for this help. Typically, this detox occurs in the liver. Your blood naturally gets filtered 20 times every day by passing through the liver. But, after a long winter or a busy stretch at work, your liver could be sending you signals to do a detox.

Physical Signs
One of the most common signs of needing a detox is gastrointestinal problems. These could include gas, bloating, or constipation and diarrhea. An uptick in allergies or headaches could also be a sign from your liver that you have excess toxins in your body.

Emotional Signs
If you notice yourself becoming more irritable or get angry quicker than typical, these are both signs to detox. Indecisiveness or general brain fog is another big sign. If you do start to notice any of these signs, you can try new at home remedies to help get your body back to normal.

At Home Detox
By adding simple foods or drinks to your diet, you can help reset your liver and get your body back on track. Not only will these help you get rid of excess toxins, but they could also give you the added benefit of weight loss as well! All the following are things you most likely already have in your pantry and could be an easy way to help your body get back on track.

Lemons
Found in 1941 by a naturopath, by combining lemons with cayenne pepper and Madal Bal, a tree syrup, you could help your body not only detoxify but also lose quite a bit of weight. One person who tried this detox even found they had lost 5 pounds in just three days! By getting rid of this extra weight, your liver will also be able to more effectively cleanse your blood in the future.

Apple Cider Vinegar
This simple kitchen staple has exploded recently with health benefits. By drinking a few tablespoons diluted with water three times per day, has been shown in some trials to aid in weight loss, regulating blood sugars and blood pressure, and help to kickstart a new, healthier lifestyle.

Tea

Tea has long been known as a health drink with many benefits. Cleansing your body is one of them! Depending on your tea blend, you could tailor it to your own needs. Adding elements like licorice or sweet anise could curb your sugar cravings while adding chamomile could help your body unwind at night for a better night's sleep. Both added benefits can help your body get back to normal as well!

Conclusion

All in all, the occasional cleanse could help your body to get back on track for a healthy lifestyle. By watching for signs that your liver needs some help, you can better know when to use a detox. With simple at home remedies, you are on your way to living a better life!

Unlocking the Secrets of the Healthiest Vinegar

Many people seem to forget that some of the healthiest foods and ingredients are normal staples in their pantry. Vinegar has many uses both in cooking and daily household chores. But there is one vinegar that has many hidden health benefits that could be the key to unlocking a healthier, more balanced lifestyle. Read here to learn how apple cider vinegar could change your life for the better.

Healthier Organs

This special vinegar acts like a tonic and antioxidant in your body. This works throughout your internal organs helping them in various ways. By working to help clear toxins from your body, apple cider vinegar helps to keep your liver and lymph nodes in a proper working state. Apple cider vinegar also helps to balance your pH levels, which can stimulate both bowel and cardiovascular function. With better bowel function, your body will be even more efficient at eliminating waste and toxins. Also, in addition to the stimulated heart activity, the acidity in the vinegar also helps to keep your triglycerides balanced and has been shown to reduce your LDL, or bad cholesterol. Lowering this LDL helps to keep your heart healthy and your veins and arteries free from clogging plaque.

Healthier Weight

To continue with keeping your insides healthy, apple cider vinegar has been shown in many studies to keep your blood sugars regulated. By slowing the rate at which your body digests carbohydrates, your insulin has more time to break down the carbohydrates, helping to keep your blood sugars balanced, even after a high carb meal. This slower digestion rate also helps to keep you feeling fuller longer and stops additional cravings for more starchy or sugary carbs. As a side effect to longer satiety, you will end up not just eating less, but also eating far fewer sugars, which could help lead to weight loss.

Healthier Hair and Skin

Lastly, in today's day and age, it is just as important to stay healthy on the outside as it is on the inside. Apple cider vinegar has been shown to have many benefits for both your skin and hair. First off, apple cider vinegar has more potassium than other kinds of vinegar. This potassium helps to topically reduce inflammation, which will stop the pain and itching due to bug bites or poison ivy. Secondly, as stated before, this household staple balances your pH levels. In addition to the precious benefits, better pH helps to keep your skin smooth, hydrated, and wrinkle free! Lastly, apple cider vinegar works at the molecular level of your hair to help keep your hair shiny and healthy. As many hair products are alkaline, they risk raising the pH of your hair, which apple cider vinegar is perfect for combating. Balancing the chemical levels in your hair will allow it to grow stronger, so your hair is shinier and easier to manage.

Overall, apple cider vinegar has many hidden benefits. By working both inside your body and out, this simple household staple can help you live a healthier, more balanced life.

ACV – The New All-Natural Anti-Dandruff Shampoo?

Many people struggle with dandruff, whether due to dry skin or bad hair products. With so many people trying to hide these annoying white flakes, many shampoos and other hair care products have labeled themselves specifically to treat this problem. But what exactly is dandruff, and are there more natural ways to combat this annoying problem? This article takes a closer look at both questions, including a newfound miracle that you probably already have sitting in your kitchen cabinet!

What is Dandruff?

Dandruff, while not serious, can be quite annoying. Typically caused by dry skin, small white, oily flakes of skin can start to fall from your hair and on your clothes. This can also cause itchiness of your scalp. During the winter, when the air outside is drier, some people do see an increase in dandruff due to their skin also drying out.

Because most people don't like having these white flakes falling on their clothes, they tend to turn to over the counter shampoos and other treatments. However, it has been noticed that there is a more natural way to help combat this problem, and most people already have this in their kitchen cupboards!

Naturally Treating Dandruff With ACV

In recent years, doctors have been harnessing the acidic power of Apple Cider Vinegar to help combat many health concerns. In addition to helping with weight loss diets, this miracle ingredient has been shown to help stop those annoying flakes from returning. As many commercialized hair care products are chemically alkaline, or basic, they can raise the pH of your scalp. By continuing to use store-bought shampoos and conditioners, this problem could continue to worsen, as there is nothing acidic to bring your pH levels back into balance. That's precisely where apple cider vinegar comes into play. As vinegar is naturally acidic, it can help restore your natural chemical levels to help stop the dryness and flaking of your scalp. But why does it need to be specifically apple cider vinegar?

In addition to its natural acidity, apple cider vinegar offers both anti-inflammatory and antimicrobial properties as well as working as an exfoliant. By helping to exfoliate your scalp, some of the excess flakes will be washed off during a shower instead of falling off onto your clothing. The anti-inflammatory helps to keep your skin calm and healthy while the antimicrobial keeps problem causing bacteria at bay.

Conclusion for Using ACV for Dandruff

As dandruff is more of an annoyance than a serious health problem, most people turn to over the counter remedies. However, the best, all-natural treatment could be as far as a short walk to your kitchen. By helping to balance the basic pH of your hair, caused by typical hair care products, apple cider vinegar can help to keep your scalp's chemical levels in check. By also helping to exfoliate the skin on your scalp and offering anti-inflammatory and antimicrobial benefits, this miracle ingredient could be the secret home remedy to keeping those annoying white flakes from ever coming back.

What Are the Benefits of ACV for My Dog?

By Samuel Turner*

Apple Cider Vinegar (referred to as ACV In this article) has been a popular home remedy for generations as a first-aid treatment. ACV may be beneficial for topical applications, including muscle aches and bruises, windburn, abrasions, sunburn, insect bites, stings, and hair care.

Over the past few years, it has been discovered that it has as many benefits for our canine family as well. Frequently reported benefits include better mobility in older dogs, reduced flea populations, enhanced skin, and coat condition, less itching and scratching, the exclusion of tear stains on the face, fewer brown or yellow urine spots on lawns, and an improvement in overall health.

A tablespoon of apple cider vinegar and honey a day could be enough to show visible improvements in the quality of your dog's skin and fur. Before applying ACV topically do a patch test on the skin and coat first, and especially if your canine is a puppy.

ACV May Be Used for Muscle Sprains in Dogs

If you find that your dog has any of the following discomforts such as sore muscles, sore paws, bruises or abrasions, apply ACV to the affected area with cotton wool or a sponge.

ACV May Be Used for Skin and Coat Treatments

After you have washed your dog, you can add one cup of ACV to the final rinse of water. Experiment with different dilutions, we recommend 1 cup of vinegar diluted in 2 to 4 cups of water.

For skin irritations, rough skin, calluses, and sunburn apply ACV (full-strength or diluted), it can be in a spray form or may be applied with cotton or a sponge.

For itchy skin and hot spots, spray with ACV. Monitor the dog to see if redness or irritation develops, if it does wash off with water and discontinue use. This might be because of a sensitive skin in the puppy or dog.

ACV May Be Used for Itchy Feet or Ears

Soaking the paws in diluted/full-strength ACV can reduce itchy feet (contracted by seasonal allergies – pollen exposure).

Place a few drops of ACV or a vinegar-based herbal tincture in each ear and gently massage, (may be applied with a cotton swab) to clean the dog's ears and to keep them healthy.

ACV May Be Used as An Insect Repellent and Flea Dip

ACV may be sprayed onto the dog's coat (tail, underbelly, neck, and torso – avoid the mouth, eyes, and nose) as it repels insects.

Pour, spray or sponge the dog or puppy entirely with ACV avoiding the mouth, nose, and eyes. Let it soak in for a few minutes, before washing the dog or puppy with a gentle shampoo.

ACV May Be Used to Clean Pet Stains and Odors

Mix 1 part of ACV with 3 parts water, pour onto stained area and blot with a paper towel, do not rub.

Pet bedding may be refreshed and deodorized by spraying it with ACV or by adding it to laundry when washing the bedding.

Pet toys can also be sprayed lightly with ACV to clean and disinfect them, just make sure they are wiped clean afterward.

Get the Most from ACV – Make Your Own

We've all heard the old adage: "an apple a day keeps the doctor away". Turns out, like so many other old wives' tales, this one has more than a grain of truth in it. And Apple Cider Vinegar (ACV) – a vinegar made from apples, sugar and yeast that our grandmothers and great-grandmothers used as a food preservative, as well as in salad dressings, marinades, vinaigrettes and chutneys because is so flavorsome and zesty – appears to have benefits that go beyond its use as a kitchen staple.

In recent years, there has been increasing interest in the health benefits of ACV. As a home remedy, it has been used to treat a wide range of complaints from varicose veins to sore throats. More recently, there has been considerable research into its ability to help with weight loss, assist with sugar control for diabetics, and improve heart health. Because of the antioxidant properties in polyphenols – a chemical found in vinegar – there have been several studies to try and determine whether apple cider vinegar could also help to prevent or reduce your risk of developing cancer. So far, the results are inconclusive.

Most people make use of store-bought ACV brands. Many of these are pasteurized, and this may result in many of the benefits inherent in ACV our ancestors loved and trusted being lost in the manufacturing process. In addition, if the ACV is packaged in plastic, you may find that the acid in the liquid causes the plastic chemicals to leach into the vinegar.

If you are going to buy apple cider vinegar at the store, you should make a point of only buying it when it is packaged in glass.

Far better, however, would be to buy raw or unpasteurized apple cider vinegar. This is not cheap – and you'll probably be paying for a whole lot of water used to dilute the vinegar.

So, why not buy a whole lot of fresh apple, and make your own. It's not difficult – if you have access to raw, fresh apples, why not make your own. In fact, you don't even have to use whole apples. There's nothing to stop you using the scraps – cores, stems, and seeds – left over from making your apple pie (or whatever) that you were going to throw into the compost (or into the garbage!).

Making apple cider vinegar is not much different to making any other fermented beverage. There are many recipes for making ACV available on the internet. A good tip, however, is to use a selection of different apples, if you can. Mix and match the proportions to come up with a flavor that suits your taste buds. For example, you could use 50% sweet apples (like Golden Delicious or Fuji); 30% sharp tasting apples (Granny Smith, McIntosh) and 20% bitter tasting apples (Dolgos crab apples or Newtown for example). However, you can use whatever apples you are able to get your hands on.

It can take three to four weeks for your raw ACV to get to the right taste. However, once it has fermented, you will have a pure source of ACV at your fingertips – or in your pantry – just as nature intended.

ACV – Liquid Gold in a Bottle?

What do you think of when you see a bottle of apple cider vinegar (ACV) on the shelf in your local supermarket – or health food store? Weight loss? Detoxification? Blood glucose control? Heart health? Cancer prevention? Skin care? There has been a surge of interest in this folk remedy in recent years as a versatile health elixir.

However, did you know that your bottle (a glass bottle to prevent plastic chemical contamination), can help you keep you healthy not only inside, but outside too?

Here are 11 uses for ACV you probably didn't know about (3):

Hair conditioner/rinse. A final rinse of your hair using half a tablespoon of ACV in one cup of water will leave hair shiny, removing any unwanted chemical residue such as chlorine.

Skin toner. Great for people with oily skin, acne, scars and age/dark spots. Dilute ACV in water in a ratio of 1:2 (or weaker if you have sensitive skin) and apply directly to clean skin twice a day. Keep it away from your eyes.

Wart remover. Soak a cotton pad in ACV and keep this in place on the wart overnight (using a band-aid or porous skin tape). Repeat this daily until the wart turns black and falls off.

Mouthwash: can help treat bad breath resulting from thrush, chronic gum infections, and tooth stains. Put 2 teaspoons into a quarter cup of water, swish around your mouth a few times and spit (or swallow if you want to). Remember to brush your teeth as the acid in ACV may damage the enamel on your teeth if left in place.

Foot fungus treatment. Dilute one part ACV to two parts water and soak your feet in it. Be prepared for some stinging if you have any sores or cuts, but it will help to kill off any fungal infections like athlete's foot. If you have a persistent infection, consider soaking your stocks in the solution and wearing them overnight (covered in a plastic bag to prevent you soaking your bed).

Body odor control. Believe it or not, a diluted (1:2) solution of ACV will help to keep you smelling fresh and clean. Simply dab the solution on your underarms instead of using a deodorant. However, it is not an antiperspirant, so you may have to reapply if you sweat a lot.

Bites and stings. Dabbing the bite or sting with undiluted ACV will help reduce the pain and irritation. It works well for jellyfish stings too.

Cleaning. Make a solution of one part ACV to nine parts water and use it to clean any surface. If you like, you can put it in a spray bottle to make cleaning easier. Simply spray on and wipe off. Undiluted, ACV also makes a great toilet, bath and shower cubicle disinfectant.

Weed killer. Spray undiluted ACV onto garden weeds such as dandelions. A great way to kill them without resorting to unhealthy chemicals.

Animal repellent Rats, mice, rabbits – or even that pesky cat that's using your flower beds as a sandbox – can be kept at bay. For the rodents, scatter a few cotton balls soaked in ACV around the house and flower beds. For cats, spray undiluted ACV along the edge of the flower beds.

Flea fighter. Dilute ACV into a 1:1 solution and apply to your dog's fur to keep fleas away. Test it on a small part of your dog's skin first to ensure he does not react badly to it.

Are the Health Benefits of ACV Real or Hype?

Now here's the thing about Apple Cider Vinegar (ACV). For decades – and probably even centuries – it has been ascribed almost magical properties to cure virtually all ailments and prevent a great many more. Alright – that is something of an exaggeration – but it is one substance that has been recommended for a startlingly wide range of uses, from combating obesity to body odors.

Cynics – and many scientists – however, put ACV's purported health benefits down to folklore and old wives' tales. In fact, some claim that taking the liquid on a regular basis could be downright dangerous, eroding your teeth enamel, churning up your insides, and worse.

So, what's the truth behind ACV? Is it good for you? Is it bad for you? Is it no more than a whimsical, centuries-old myth?

The clearest answer we could find it that there is no clear answer at all.

Let's look at one of the most held beliefs about ACV – that it assists with weight loss. There are studies that have found that ACV (and vinegar, in general, may reduce the absorption of starches and slow digestion, which helps to make one feel full. There is also a study that shows that helps to keep blood sugar level in check to some extent overnight. Both these phenomena help to suppress appetite. But does that translate into weight loss?

What about claims that ACV helps with the management of diabetes because of its positive effects on blood glucose control? As mentioned, there are studies that indicate that ACV does influence blood glucose – in mice. But so far, these results have not been repeated in large, controlled human studies. Clearly, more research is required.

What about heart disease and cancer, two areas where ACV consumption is said to possibly have some positive benefits.

Animal studies, as well as lab-based studies on cells, have indicated that vinegar – and therefore probably ACV – have some anti-cancer effects. However, the results in observational human studies have been contradictory, with one study indicating a decrease in cancer, and another an increase.

There was some excitement after the results of a human trial that showed that vinegar consumption results in a reduction in triglycerides (the stuff that leads to clogged up arteries) were published in 2009. However, in the almost decade since, no other studies have been able to replicate these results. To be fair, there have not any studies performed that examine the effects of regular vinegar consumption on cardiovascular events or mortality; but one study involving diabetics revealed no change in their blood fat content after eight weeks of daily ACV consumption.

7 Things You Thought You Knew About Apple Cider Vinegar That Are Not True

By Samuel Turner*

Over the last couple of years, there has been a lot of hype regarding the numerous benefits of apple cider vinegar. However, a large amount of the benefits that are touted by the media about apple cider vinegar are not necessarily the truth. In this article, we will be looking at some of these things that you may believe about apple cider vinegar.

It Is A Quick Fix for Weight Loss

Most people who use apple cider vinegar daily do so because they believe that it will help them lose a large amount of weight very quickly. However, this may not be entirely true. Although it can help you lose a significant amount of weight it is not the quick fix that some people would have you believe it is.

It Will Get Rid of Diabetes

Sadly, drinking a few glasses of apple cider vinegar daily will not cure your diabetes. Apple cider vinegar does help to stabilize your blood sugars for a short period of time, but it will not mean the end of your condition.

No More Cholesterol

Although there has been a significant amount of research that indicates the use of apple cider vinegar will reduce the amount of cholesterol in your bloodstream. However, most of this research only consists out of animal studies. Until more research is completed on the effect of apple cider vinegar on cholesterol in humans it cannot be taken as a fact that it could improve your cholesterol levels.

It is Entirely Safe to Use

When you first investigate the benefits of using apple cider vinegar daily you may be fooled into thinking that it is safe to use, and you will not experience any side effects. However, using a large amount of apple cider vinegar daily could have significant effects on your health. Apple cider vinegar has been linked with damage to the enamel on your teeth as well as damage to your digestive system.

It is A Miracle Cure for Your Gut

There is denying that apple cider vinegar has an impact on your digestive system. Unfortunately, it may not always be a positive impact. There has been significant research which seems to indicate that using large amounts of apple cider vinegar can make the symptoms of certain digestive conditions significantly worse. It is especially dangerous for individuals who suffer from gastroparesis.

It Is Anticarcinogenic

Much of the information available about apple cider vinegar seems to indicate that apple cider vinegar has the potential to destroy all cancer cells present in your body. However, there is no concrete evidence that proves that this is the truth.

It is Only Meant for Eating

Many people believe that the only way to use apple cider vinegar is by drinking it. However, there are dozens of other uses for this vinegar. It makes an excellent all-purpose cleaner and you can even use it to tone your skin.

Can ACV Control Fleas on Your Pet?

As a pet owner, there is nothing more irritating than having to deal with an infestation of fleas. These annoying parasitic bugs are the carriers of a variety of diseases. Additionally, they cause unbearable itching and irritation. It is important to get control of the infection as soon as possible, however, most of us are concerned about all the chemicals in conventional pest control medicine. Would you believe that one of the most effective pest killers is probably in your kitchen cupboard at this moment?

How Does It Work?

You may be quite surprised to learn that apple cider vinegar does not actually cause the fleas on your pet to die. However, the highly acidic nature of this vinegar causes extreme discomfort to these pests. Although you can use apple cider vinegar to effectively treat an infestation of fleas it is far more effective if you use it to prevent your pet from becoming infected in the first place. Apple cider vinegar is a great option for pet care as it is safe for animals and children and it is unlikely to cause any irritation to your pet. It is important to choose a safe and natural option for flea and pest control because most commercial flea repellent products contain dangerous chemicals that are harmful to both you and your pet.

How Should I Use It?

When you first learn about the amazing properties of apple cider vinegar you may feel the urge to dip your dog into a large vat of this vinegar. However, this is not likely to be very effective. Instead, consider adding some apple cider vinegar to your pets drinking water. However, it is always important to dilute the vinegar before you give it to your pet to ensure that it does not damage the enamel on their teeth or their delicate digestive systems. Another way to use apple cider vinegar on your pet is to make a solution that your spray onto your pet's coat. The solution should contain equal parts of water and apple cider vinegar. Then when you notice any fleas on your pet you should begin spraying their coats once every day. You can also add a few drops of essential oils to your spray to make it even more effective. Lavender oil and cedar oil are particularly effective for reducing pests on your animals.

Other Home Remedies

One of the most effective home remedies for getting rid of fleas on your pet is essential oils. lemongrass, cedarwood, peppermint, rosemary, and thyme are essential oils that are particularly good at warding off pests. Dilute eight to ten drops of essential oils in a little water and place the solution on the back of your pets' neck below the collar. Just take care never to use tea tree oil on your animals as it is highly toxic to them. Alternatively, you can add the juice of half a lemon to your pets drinking water to ward off ticks and fleas.

8 Amazing Life Hacks with Apple Cider Vinegar

Apple Cider Vinegar (ACV) has been used for thousands of years as a natural remedy for ailments. That's right, something that's been sitting in your pantry for who knows how long, offers tremendous health benefits. But not only that, it can be used in a variety of ways for a vast range of things. Check out our exciting list of life hacks with ACV!

1. Natural Detergent

ACV is known for its antibacterial properties. Consequently, it can be used to clean countertops, appliances, and other household items. Simply mix 1 part ACV with 1 part water, pour it into a spray bottle, and voila; you now have your very own cost-effective natural detergent.

2. Odor Repellent

Beyond its bacteria-fighting effects, it can neutralize off-putting scents. While it may not smell appealing, to begin with, its pH levels will eliminate nasty smelling bacteria. Place a little in a dish or Tupperware to get rid of the unwelcome smell.

3. Reducing Risk of Diabetes

Studies show that this substance can improve insulin sensitivity. Insulin is an essential hormone that regulates blood sugar levels. In saying so, ACV can prevent sugar spikes and insulin resistance that may lead to type 2 diabetes.

4. Wart Remover

A trip to the doctor can be costly, painful, and ineffective at times. If you wish to opt for a more sustainable solution to warts, then consider plastering ACV on your wart with cotton wool. The high acidic profile of the substance will burn off the wart.

5. Weight Loss

Research suggests that it prevents the digestion of starch and suppresses appetite. As a result, it reduces the number of calories absorbed into the body and combats overeating. While this may not encourage weight loss optimally, it will prevent steady weight gain. Drink a combination of 1 part ACV and 3 parts water to reap the benefits. Use this alongside a healthy diet and exercise for maximum fat burning potential.

6. Dandruff Remedy

A common cause of dandruff is the accumulation of excess yeast on the scalp. ACV has a high acidic profile; therefore, it creates an environment in which yeast cannot grow. This will prevent this common cause of dandruff and may combat it all together.

7. Skin Cleanser

Its antibacterial properties are not limited to household detergents. In the right concentrations, it can effectively reduce skin conditions and blemishes. ACV's pH balance supports the skin's protective acid mantle. Consequently, it ensures that external aggressors do not damage the skin. Furthermore, the high acidity content works as a natural exfoliator. This removes dead skin cells and encourages the growth of new ones.

8. Juice

Many of its benefits pertain to the role it plays inside the body. Therefore, consuming it is one of the most effective ways to reap the rewards of weight loss and blood sugar control. While the flavor is distinct and not for everyone, adding it to a blended juice will give it a surprisingly delightful tang. Plus, you will be enriched with the added health benefits.

What's So Great About Apple Cider Vinegar?

From "miracle cure" to "magic elixir", Apple Cider Vinegar (ACV) is said to contain unprecedented healing properties. The popular household product has, for many years, found its way into delightful dishes and/or been used as a detergent. However, many people are not completely aware of the health potential this product has. Numerous studies have been and continue to be done in order to shed light on the ways in which ACV effects the body. For the most part, these studies show increasingly positive results. They serve as evidence supporting the consumption of ACV in boosting your quality of life. They also substantiate the extensive and often overwhelming marketing of ACV as an ultimate health remedy. But, in order to fully understand its role in the body we need to take a closer look at it. In this article, we will outline the benefits of consuming it and possible risks. We will determine whether it is as great as claims make it out to be.

It Reduces the Risk of Heart Disease and Diabetes

One of the most prominent and well-documented roles that it plays in the body is lowering blood sugar levels. As a result, it can minimize the risk of heart disease and diabetes. Studies suggest that ACV inhibits digestive enzymes that break down starch in the body. The resulting effect is that the undigested starch reduces an individual's blood sugar (glycemic) response. Conversely to a high glycemic response, a low one decreases the likelihood of blood sugar spikes and subsequent cardiovascular strain. Furthermore, ACV may improve insulin sensitivity. Insulin is a hormone responsible for regulating blood sugar levels. People that suffer from type 2 diabetes have insulin imbalances. Hence, ACV's role in supporting insulin sensitivity reduces one's risk of type 2 diabetes as it maintains proper functioning. To read more about this, you can access the full publication here.

It Supports Digestion and Boosts Immune Strength

The fact that ACV prevents the digestion of starch has several additional benefits. For one, it is said to work as a prebiotic. The undigested starch serves as a source of nutrition for healthy bacteria. This stimulates the growth of probiotics which maintain optimal digestive health. This is because probiotics inhibit the detrimental effects of bad bacteria. Furthermore, this will support immune strength. As a result of the consumption of ACV, your body receives better nutrition and can fight off illness more effectively.

It Encourages Weight Loss

One of the most appealing benefits of ACV is its ability to promote fat burning. Acetic acid, the main component of ACV, promotes fat oxidation and prevents the absorption of calories. As a result, it may encourage the body's fat burning capacity. A study conducted in Japan supports these notions. There are, however, some concerns regarding this benefit. For one, results are said to be extremely slow and happen over a lengthy period. In essence, the consumption of ACV may support weight loss but should be used alongside a balanced diet and frequent exercise.

But Are There Concerns?

Acetic acid is found in most vinegar products. Therefore, the benefits are not exclusive to Apple Cider Vinegar.

"Mother of vinegar", a beneficial substance found after the fermentation process, is often filtered out of shop-bought products.

Due to its acidic nature, ACV may lead to burns and/or erosion if consumed excessively.

There you have it, a few reasons why ACV is a must-have product and a few of the concerns to look out for. Ultimately, ACV may support your overall health in combination with balanced lifestyle habits. Now go on and get your own ACV to start reaping the rewards today!

Is Apple Cider Vinegar Considered A Superfood?

Superfoods are all the hype. From almonds to coconut oil, health-conscious consumers are looking to superfoods as a natural way of remedying health problems. Every now and then a new superfood pops up in the limelight because of claims that it will solve all your problems. Today, Apple Cider Vinegar is gaining increasing recognition as being the key to a more fruitful life. But is it as good as these claims suggest? Does it live up to the hype? In this article, we will provide more information about this popular product and the health benefits it may have. In doing so, you can make wiser consumer choices the next time you visit the grocery store.

What is ACV?

Before we can look at the health benefits, it is important to understand what ACV is. In short, it is a by-product of a fermentation process between apples and sugar. During the fermentation process, good bacteria feed off the sugars to form ethanol. The main role of this bacteria is to convert the ethanol into acetic acid. Acetic acid, which is the main component of ACV, is the ingredient that is said to deliver the wonderful benefits. ACV is not a new product. It has been around for centuries and forms an intrinsic part of traditional healing practices. However, recently it is gaining popularity because of the many surfacing studies.

What Are the Health Claims?

1) Supports Weight Loss

Evidence suggests that consuming ACV directly impacts bodily functions necessary for burning fat. They state that acetic acid's ability to block the digestion of starch is a key contributing factor. This is because it reduces the rate at which the body absorbs calories and stores fat. However, further studies report that the fat burning potential is very low. In saying so, ACV may be used alongside a conscious eating plan and exercise to deliver optimal results. Another weight loss supporting benefit is its ability to suppress an individual's appetite. As a result, it can prevent weight gain from overeating.

2) Reduces Blood Sugar Levels

As we have mentioned, ACV inhibits the digestion of heavy starch. Beyond the weight loss potential, this can lead to reduced blood sugar levels. Furthermore, it has been shown to positively affect insulin sensitivity. Hence, inhibit insulin resistance. This means that insulin will properly regulate blood sugar levels. By keeping levels low, acetic acid can prevent sugar spikes and cardiovascular disease. However, this applies to all vinegar products containing it. Not just Apple Cider Vinegar. In saying so, it may prove beneficial but is not the only option available.

3) Rich in Potassium

In short, ACV does not contain high quantities of potassium. Especially in comparison with other produce. ACV generally contains 11mg of potassium per serving. The recommended dietary intake is between 2800mg and 3800mg per day. Therefore, you would need to drink a substantial amount. This is not a great idea as the highly acidic profile of it may lead to adverse side effects.

Is Drinking It Worth It?

The reasons to consume it are not completely compelling. This is because there is still a lot of research to be done and what we do know is very limited. There are most certainly benefits of drinking it, however, one cannot completely rely on it to deliver optimal health effects. Consuming ACV should be done alongside a well-curated meal plan and exercise.

Are the Claims About Apple Cider Vinegar True?

By Danielle Sanders*

Apple Cider Vinegar (ACV), a product that can be found in most US homes, has been used as a natural remedy for centuries. Many people claim that it offers powerful health benefits. From preventing dandruff to encouraging weight loss, this "miracle food" has become increasingly popular over the years. But is there any truth in these statements? Are there any false reports? In this article, we outline whether ACV can live up to some of the bolder claims about its benefits.

It can whiten teeth and/or dentures

ACV does not clean or whiten teeth/dentures. In fact, an expert was shocked to hear about this report. When asked by CNN whether there was any truth in this claim, she stated that "Cleaning dentures or rinsing with vinegar is not a good idea. It too could put your teeth at risk." She attributes this comment to the fact that the extremely high acidity of it can damage the teeth's enamel. Enamel is a protective coating that prevents bacteria from forming cavities.

It can reduce blood sugar levels

While there aren't any conclusive reports, there is a substantial amount of evidence linking ACV to reduced blood sugar levels. The claims are substantiated by the fact that vinegar blocks the digestion of starch. As a result, starchy foods will be less likely to cause sugar spikes and subsequent heart problems. Furthermore, ACV is said to improve insulin sensitivity. Insulin, a hormone that regulates blood sugar, imbalances can lead to type 2 diabetes. In saying so, ACV may serve as a preventative measure and help combat cardiovascular disease from high blood sugar.

It can support weight loss

There is some truth in this statement, although, it will not be as effective as various other methods. For example, ACV's role in inhibiting starch digestion has an impact on the body's fat burning potential. For one, it reduces the number of calories absorbed into the body. Furthermore, it suppresses an individual's appetite. Consequently, it may prevent overeating and subsequent weight gain.

It can combat dandruff

This claim is true. A common cause of dandruff is yeast growth on the scalp. However, the high acidity profile of ACV interacts with the scalp's pH level. Consequently, it creates an environment in which yeast is not conducive. If you are wanting to concoct your own anti-dandruff shampoo using ACV, then click here.

It can remedy an aggravated throat

There is truth in this claim. Often, germs are unable to survive and thrive within a highly acidic environment. ACV creates such an environment; thus, it can eliminate harmful germs. This will ultimately minimize the impact of a sore throat. However, it is not the optimal remedy in comparison to clinically proven medication. Consumers should gargle an ACV mixture as soon as they experience any pain.

It can alleviate pain

Unfortunately, beyond a sore throat, ACV cannot relieve severe pain. Many believe that beta-carotene, found in it, can fight free radicals. However, the Arthritis Foundation state that the quantity is so small it will not have any effect. Therefore, it is highly unlikely that it can prevent pain-inducing free radicals.

Is Acne Preventable Using Apple Cider Vinegar?

Apple Cider Vinegar (ACV) has grown in popularity over the years because of claims that it can benefit the body. So much so that it is subject to major health-conscious consuming discussions. There are many studies aiming to prove these benefits. While many of them are not conclusive, they do suggest that it promotes weight loss and lowers blood sugar levels to name a few. Today we will focus on whether it can cure acne and if you should consider using it.

Bacteria Fighting Properties

Studies suggest that ACV is a natural antibacterial. More specifically, it is shown to reduce bacteria by 90% in certain subjects. Acne, an inflammatory skin condition that causes severe pimples and spots, is often a result of Propionibacterium acnes. Propionibacterium acnes, or P. acnes, is a specific strain of bacteria that leads to the condition. While research pertaining to ACV's ability to fight these specific bacteria are inconclusive, its antibacterial properties bode well for its effectiveness. Furthermore, the substances found within ACV (acetic, citric, lactic and succinic acid) have seen some positive research in fighting P. acnes. In saying so, it may provide relief from acne, but more evidence pertaining to its direct influence is needed.

Ability to Reduce Scarring

Skin discoloration and scarring are common side effects of acne. ACV may help remedy these concerns. The application of it to the skin is known as chemical peeling. This is a process whereby the acids in the solution exfoliate the outer layers of the skin and promote the development of healthy new cells. Succinic and Lactic Acid has been shown to reduce inflammation and improve pigmentation respectively. As a result, they may remedy scarring. That said, further research into ACV's role in providing these effects is necessary to make a conclusive claim.

It May Cause Burns

ACV has a highly acidic profile. Although bacteria are not conducive to the environment that it creates, the skin may suffer as well. For instance, frequent contact with high concentrations of ACV can cause burns. While it is unlikely that you will lather yourself in it, the concern needs to be considered. One should never apply it to open wounds and, in the case of sensitive skin, dilute it with water.

In Conclusion

The specific acids found within ACV have been shown to reduce symptoms of acne. Furthermore, they may also prevent common side effects of the condition. This bodes well for its use as an effective remedy for the condition. However, one needs to know use is not void of negative side effects. Precaution should be taken before application and results may significantly vary across individuals.

Method

Combine 1 part ACV with 3 parts water.

Clean the face with organic face wash and lightly dry.

Apply the ACV mixture to the skin using cotton.

Let it sit for approximately 20 seconds before rinsing off and drying. You should rinse sooner if you experience burning sensations.

This process can be done 1 – 2 times per day. You should not exceed this recommendation as too much contact with it can lead to painful side effects.

How to Make Your Own Apple Cider Vinegar

Apple Cider Vinegar (ACV) is a miracle product. It offers tremendous health benefits and adds a delightful tang to dishes. If you are a fan of this vinegar but conscious of your health, then you may want to consider making your own. This homemade ACV recipe is exceptionally easy to follow, and the resulting product will not contain any questionable ingredients. Hence, you can enjoy the distinguished flavor without worrying about potential side effects. Continue reading for the recipe to this healthy homemade ACV.

What You'll Need:

A large, glass jar (a half gallon mason jar will work best)

Cheesecloth

An elastic band to secure the cheesecloth to the jar

A glass weight (this will keep the apples below the water's surface)

Fresh, organic apples

Filtered water

2 – 3 tablespoons of raw cane sugar per half gallon jar.

Step 1 – Prepping Your ACV

Prepping your area – Clean your utensils, jar, and countertops with warm, soapy water. Let everything air-dry before assembling. Properly cleaning your workspace will ensure that bad bacteria is not present during the fermentation process.

Prepping your apples – Rinse your apples in cold water and wipe off any dirt and/or residue. As a rule of thumb, use unbruised apples. If you only have bruised or blemished ones, then cut off these unappealing bits.

Tip: You can use whole, diced apples or only the apple skins for this Apple Cider Vinegar.

Step 2 – Assembling Your ACV

Toss your clean, diced apples or apple skins into the mason jar until it is ¾ full.

Pour the filtered water into the jar until the apples are fully covered. Sprinkle over the sugar. The sugar is a source of food for beneficial bacteria, allowing the fermentation process to take place. Beneficial bacteria offer many nutritional benefits.

You will need a glass fermentation weight to submerge the apples below the water. If you can't get a hold of one, then you will need to get a little creative. Many people use a clean zip-lock bag filled with water and a sterilized rock. Ensure that your weight submerges all the apples and that no parts are exposed to the air. This can encourage the growth of mold which will spoil your ACV.

Secure a doubled-up piece of cheesecloth to the top of the jar with an elastic band. This will keep fruit flies and other bugs out of your concoction.

Step 3 – Letting It Ferment

Stash your mixture, away from direct sunlight, in a room-temperature environment (approximately 70°F). Anywhere colder will make the fermentation process take longer. Leave it to ferment for 4 weeks.

If, after 3 days, little bubbles start to form then the process is working! This is an indication that the beneficial bacteria are converting the sugars into CO_2.

Check on your brew every couple of days to make sure that the apples are still submerged. The soon-to-be ACV may smell sweet in the beginning; however, it will start to smell sourer as the process takes place.

Step 4 – Straining & Storing Your ACV

A substance called "mother" may form on the top of the jar. This is a sign that the fermentation process is underway. This substance can be stored in a jar with ACV to be used as a starter culture for your next batch!

After 4 weeks, your ACV will be ready to strain. Remove your weight and squeeze out as much of the apples as possible using a cheesecloth.

Pour the strained liquid back into the jar and cover with the cheesecloth. Leave the ACV to ferment for a further 2 – 3 weeks, stirring every other day.

Taste the ACV after the second fermentation. If you are happy with the taste, then bottle and seal it. Start enjoying your home-made Apple Cider Vinegar in a variety of exciting ways!

Unlocking the Secrets of the Healthiest Vinegar

Many people seem to forget that some of the healthiest foods and ingredients are normal staples in their pantry. Vinegar has many uses both in cooking and daily household chores. But there is one vinegar that has many hidden health benefits that could be the key to unlocking a healthier, more balanced lifestyle. Read here to learn how apple cider vinegar could change your life for the better.

Healthier Organs

This special vinegar acts a tonic and antioxidant in your body. This works throughout your internal organs helping them in various ways. By working to help clear toxins from your body, apple cider vinegar helps to keep your liver and lymph nodes in a proper working state. Apple cider vinegar also helps to balance your pH levels, which can stimulate both bowel and cardiovascular function. With better bowel function, your body will be even more efficient at eliminating waste and toxins. Also, in addition to the stimulated heart activity, the acidity in the vinegar also helps to keep your triglycerides balanced and has been shown to reduce your LDL, or bad cholesterol. Lowering this LDL helps to keep your heart healthy and your veins and arteries free from clogging plaque.

Healthier Weight

To continue with keeping your insides healthy, apple cider vinegar has been shown in many studies to keep your blood sugars regulated. By slowing the rate at which your body digests carbohydrates, your insulin has more time to break down the carbohydrates, helping to keep your blood sugars balanced, even after a high carb meal. This slower digestion rate also helps to keep you feeling fuller longer and stops additional cravings for more starchy or sugary carbs. As a side effect to longer satiety, you will end up not just eating less, but also eating far fewer sugars, which could help lead to weight loss.

Healthier Hair and Skin

Lastly, in today's day and age, it is just as important to stay healthy on the outside as it is on the inside. Apple cider vinegar has been shown to have many benefits for both your skin and hair. First off, apple cider vinegar has more potassium than other kinds of vinegar. This potassium helps to topically reduce inflammation, which will stop the pain and itching due to bug bites or poison ivy. Secondly, as stated before, this household staple balances your pH levels. In addition to the precious benefits, better pH helps to keep your skin smooth, hydrated, and wrinkle free! Lastly, apple cider vinegar works at the molecular level of your hair to help keep your hair shiny and healthy. As many hair products are alkaline, they risk raising the pH of your hair, which apple cider vinegar is perfect for combating. Balancing the chemical levels in your hair will allow it to grow stronger, so your hair is shinier and easier to manage.

Overall, apple cider vinegar has many hidden benefits. By working both inside your body and out, this simple household staple can help you live a healthier, more balanced life.

In recent months, yet another diet craze has swept of the weight loss world. Many people claim drinking apple cider vinegar before meals can help kickstart your metabolism to keep those pounds off. But are these claims true, and what research exists to back these absurd claims?

Presumed Benefits

There are many ways dieters claim this miracle vinegar can help to shed excess pounds from your waistline. By stimulating digestion, your body begins to digest your food faster and get rid of excess waste, like fats, before they have a time to absorb into your body. Getting rid of the excess waste faster means less of the fat from your food is being used for energy, so your body will naturally begin to use its fat stores instead to make up for the difference. Others have stated that this vinegar helps to stimulate protein utilization. Using the proteins from food faster allows the body to create more growth hormone, which is the key to keeping a high resting metabolism rate. Lastly, because the vinegar is sourced from apples, it contains apple pectin, this pectin has been shown to act as an appetite suppressant. Taking apple cider vinegar before meals can cut down on the calories you consume in each meal. However, with all of these proclaimed weight loss benefits, there are more downsides to jumping on this food fad.

Downsides to Vinegar

Any doctor or scientist you speak to will say the number one, most important part of any new medical information is that it is will be backed by medical research. However, there is almost no research whatsoever to back these crazy claims. In fact, the European Food Safety Authority has approved zero of these claims. Without research, most people are blindly following this new trend because they heard about it through an unknown source, usually friends or the internet. Not only is using apple cider vinegar for weight loss not backed by research but drinking this as a beverage everyday can cause health problems.

High Acidity

Just like any vinegar, apple cider vinegar has a high acidity. While some acid in your diet is ok to digest, drinking too much of it can cause many health problems. Your teeth's enamel, which keeps your teeth strong and healthy can be eroded by drinking acidic drinks. Also, your throat is not made to constantly have acid in it, which can lead to erosion of your esophagus. Acid, however, is not the only problem that is caused by drinking vinegar.

Messing with Your Body's Nutrients

As apple cider vinegar does help to quicken your digestion, it does not give your body enough time to absorb the nutrients it does need to survive. Many people who have started this fad have low potassium levels. Without proper potassium, your muscles and nerves cannot properly send and receive the mental signals they need to work. Additionally, it has been shown that medications, like those to treat diabetes and heart disease are not properly absorbed when following this diet.

Conclusion

All in all, it is important to do your own research before jumping on a new diet bandwagon. With so many potential problems to adding apple cider vinegar into your daily drinks, this may be one diet to stay away from.

Apple Cider Vinegar – A Weight Loss Miracle?

In recent months, yet another diet craze has swept of the weight loss world. Many people claim drinking apple cider vinegar before meals can help kickstart your metabolism to keep those pounds off. But are these claims true, and what research exists to back these absurd claims?

Presumed Benefits

There are many ways dieters claim this miracle vinegar can help to shed excess pounds from your waistline. By stimulating digestion, your body begins to digest your food faster and get rid of excess waste, like fats, before they have a time to absorb into your body. Getting rid of the excess waste faster means less of the fat from your food is being used for energy, so your body will naturally begin to use its fat stores instead to make up for the difference. Others have stated that this vinegar helps to stimulate protein utilization. Using the proteins from food faster allows the body to create more growth hormone, which is the key to keeping a high resting metabolism rate. Lastly, because the vinegar is sourced from apples, it contains apple pectin, this pectin has been shown to act as an appetite suppressant. Taking apple cider vinegar before meals can cut down on the calories you consume in each meal. However, with all these proclaimed weight loss benefits, there are more downsides to jumping on this food fad.

Downsides to Vinegar

Any doctor or scientist you speak to will say the number one, most important part of any new medical information is that it is will be backed by medical research. However, there is almost no research whatsoever to back these crazy claims. In fact, the European Food Safety Authority has approved zero of these claims. Without research, most people are blindly following this new trend because they heard about it through an unknown source, usually friends or the internet. Not only is using apple cider vinegar for weight loss not backed by research but drinking this as a beverage everyday can cause health problems.

High Acidity

Just like any vinegar, apple cider vinegar has a high acidity. While some acid in your diet is ok to digest, drinking too much of it can cause many health problems. Your teeth's enamel, which keeps your teeth strong and healthy can be eroded by drinking acidic drinks. Also, your throat is not made to constantly have acid in it, which can lead to erosion of your esophagus. Acid, however, is not the only problem that is caused by drinking vinegar.

Messing with Your Body's Nutrients

As apple cider vinegar does help to quicken your digestion, it does not give your body enough time to absorb the nutrients it does need to survive. Many people who have started this fad have low potassium levels. Without proper potassium, your muscles and nerves cannot properly send and receive the mental signals they need to work. Additionally, it has been shown that medications, like those to treat diabetes and heart disease are not properly absorbed when following this diet.

Conclusion

All in all, it is important to do your own research before jumping on a new diet bandwagon. With so many potential problems to adding apple cider vinegar into your daily drinks, this may be one diet to stay away from.

The Pros & Cons of Apple Cider Vinegar

It is believed that apple cider vinegar can not only encourage weight loss but also increase glucose tolerance for those with type 2 diabetes, improve heart health and it can also be a treatment for dandruff. It seems to be considered as a kind of health booster, although, there may be some downfalls involved with using apple cider vinegar.

How Does Apple Cider Vinegar Work?

Apple cider vinegar starts off as apple juice that is fermented by adding yeast which converts the fruit sugar into alcohol. Bacteria then converts the alcohol into acetic acid, which is the ingredient that offers the various health benefits such as raising blood sugar levels after meals which could help to encourage weight loss when following a low-calorie diet.

According to research, it is recommended that you should use apple cider vinegar by taking one teaspoon before a meal. It can also be used by adding it to meals or drinks which may help avoid its bitter taste. This health booster can be used in detox diet plans to improve health and increase weight loss.

Available Forms of ACV to Choose From

As a result of its rapidly growing popularity, apple cider vinegar is not only available in liquid form. More recently, it is also available in a variety of different health products and even in pill form which would make use a lot more convenient.

Regardless of the convenience of using pills rather than the bitter tasting liquid, it seems that consuming the liquid would be a far better option when comparing the two. Research shows that some studies have been done to compare apple cider vinegar liquid with pills and it seems that the liquid contains between 5 and 6 percent acetic acid while the pills contain between 0.4 and 30 percent of acetic acid. This is concerning because the pills would then range from inadequate and ineffective levels of acetic acid to worrying and potentially dangerous levels.

The Concerns to Consider When Using Apple Cider Vinegar

Even though this seems like a natural weight loss aid and fantastic health booster, there are also some concerns regarding the use of apple cider vinegar according to research. Some evidence suggests that you should use apple cider vinegar with caution because of its high levels of acidity which could possibly cause some damage for your throat, teeth, and stomach. It is somewhat concerning that household products that contain more than 20% acetic acid are considered poisonous because this rule somehow does not apply to dietary supplements and foods.

Using apple cider vinegar can cause your potassium levels to drop which will negatively affect the way your muscles and nerve's function which is rather worrying. Furthermore, it may improve insulin levels for those with type 2 diabetes, it can worsen insulin levels for those with type 1 diabetes.

The Bottom Line

Apple cider vinegar does seem to yield the health benefits of boosting weight loss and improving glucose tolerance in people who suffer from diabetes, however, there is not much evidence to support that it really does work. It seems easy to incorporate the use of apple cider vinegar into your diet and there are many suggested methods available online, it can even be added into meals or mixed with drinks. It is also available in other forms, such as pill form which could be more convenient to use, although, the liquid form is far more appropriate when considering that studies show apple cider vinegar pills contain anything from ineffective to potentially dangerous levels of acetic acid.

When opting to consider the use of apple cider vinegar for weight loss, as a detox or to improve glucose tolerance, it is best to consult your healthcare practitioner prior to use to first properly establish the safety and concerns for your individual dietary requirements and ensure that it will not cause any health concerns for you.

A little something- something about me...

I have always dreamt of having a fabulous figure, just like my favorite celebrities! They have curves in all the right places, and boy, do they look amazing in anything and everything they wear.

It may sound ridiculous, but I am someone who can gain weight, even if I breathe! Yes, I have a big tendency to put on extra kilos, and that's exactly why I try and do everything possible to keep my weight in check. Because it takes a whole lot of effort to lose weight (phew!).

Last month, I had a long chat with my honey, who asked me to try apple cider vinegar for its several health benefits, including weight loss. I wasn't too sure if I should, but I decided to go ahead with the plan. After all, there's no harm in trying!

So, along with a healthy diet and an intense workout routine, apple cider vinegar became a part of my life. I dedicatedly consumed it every single day for a month, and I think it's one of my best decisions. Apart from helping me lose weight, it did a lot more.

Excited to know? Keep reading!

Apple cider vinegar is a superfood that not only lowers your blood sugar levels but can also prevent cardiovascular diseases. Image courtesy: Shutterstock

Go for the apple cider vinegar with "the mother"

Before jumping onto the apple cider vinegar bandwagon, I decided to do proper research before buying the right variant. There are a million varieties online, so you really need to know what to pick. Several blogs and health websites recommended going for apple cider vinegar "with the mother", and that's exactly what I bought!

But what exactly is it? It means that the original bacteria culture that was used to make the vinegar was not filtered out during the manufacturing process. In a nutshell, the nutrients and bacteria were not distilled after the vinegar was ready. And how do you identify it? You see brown-colored particles settled at the bottom of the bottle.

This variant of apple cider vinegar is said to help with weight loss, heart health, managing cholesterol and blood sugar levels.

My 30-day apple cider vinegar ritual

After checking with my physician, I decided to start this practice. On the very first day, I decided to go for a day-long cleanse. In a liter of water, I added two teaspoons of apple cider vinegar, and kept drinking it after every few hours. You might not like the taste in the beginning, but you will eventually get used to it.

The first day was not bad, although I kept running to the loo every now and then!

The next day onward, I began my mornings with a teaspoon of apple cider vinegar and half a teaspoon of honey, with a cup of warm water. I followed this practice every single day for a month, and here's what I observed:

Do you know that an apple cider vinegar bath is the answer to most skin concerns? I used to feel bloated all the time, but after trying ACV, I felt much lighter and active.

My skin improved and how! Since I have oily skin, I am perpetually at risk of breakouts, but this entire month, my face was visibly clear!

I felt a huge difference in my digestion, and my appetite got smaller. I feel my hunger pangs can now be easily controlled.

My cholesterol levels are stable, even though I did eat junk food in the middle (more than once).

Although my weight has not reduced drastically, I feel much lighter and healthier!

So, ladies and gentlemen, apple cider vinegar truly lives up to its hype. I did get my dream figure and I am much healthier today. One step closer to my goal, I'd say!

Summary/Conclusion

WHAT IS APPLE CIDER VINEGAR?
Have you ever stopped to ask yourself what vinegar is made from? Many people are surprised to learn that vinegar is produced through the fermentation of ethanol alcohol found in products like beer, champagne, cider, etc. During the process of fermentation, bacteria cultures break down ethanol into byproducts including acetic acid, vitamins, and minerals.

There are many kinds of vinegar including balsamic vinegar, rice vinegar, white vinegar, red wine vinegar, malt vinegar, cane vinegar, and — our favorite — apple cider vinegar. Each of these vinegars is created by adding original ingredients that create unique qualities and flavor profiles.

Homemade apple cider vinegar is made by submerging crushed apples and apple scraps in a solution of cane sugar. This begins the fermentation process that takes 3-6 weeks to complete. Find more on how to make your own ACV here.

WHAT IS APPLE CIDER VINEGAR USED FOR?

If you thought apple cider vinegar was just a pungent addition to a handful of recipes, think again. This miracle product has a wide range of uses that will have you reaching for it on the regular.

Keep your ACV handy for the following purposes:

Cleaning

Apple cider vinegar is often used as a natural alternative to harmful cleaning products. Use ACV around the house in the following ways:

-To eliminate odor: Mix ACV with water to create a deodorizing spray.

-To clean surfaces: Mix 1 part ACV with 2 parts water as an alternative to harmful cleaners.
-To catch fruit flies: Put ACV and dish soap in an open container.
-To kill weeds: Mix ACV, lemon, and soap and spray onto affected areas.
-To clean toothbrush: Mix ACV, baking soda, and water and soak toothbrush for a half hour, rinse.
-To wash dishes: Rinse dishes in ACV or add to dishwasher.

Self-Care + Hygiene

Apple cider vinegar is often used as a natural remedy for ailments and can be integrated into many self-care rituals. Try using ACV for the following:

-To calm a sore throat: Mix ACV with water and gargle to kill harmful bacteria.
-To reduce signs of aging: Mix 1 part ACV with 2 parts water to create a toner.
-To remedy skin conditions: Add 1-2 cups of ACV to a warm bath.
-To promote healthy hair: Mix equal parts ACV and water and leave in hair for 5 minutes.
-To treat dandruff: Massage equal parts ACV and water into scalp, rinse.
-To whiten teeth: Rub ACV on teeth with a cotton swab, rinse.
-To treat acne: Mix ACV and water and apply a small amount to affected areas.
-To treat warts: Apply ACV to affected areas. (Be warned that this treatment is painful).
-To prevent body odor: Mix ACV with water and wipe on the underarms.

Cooking

Apple cider vinegar can be used in cooking in many ways. Along with being a delicious addition to soup and sauce recipes, ACV can be used for the following:

-To clean fruits and vegetables: Wash in ACV to kill bacteria.
-To preserve food: Use ACV as a pickling agent.
-To make salad dressing: Mix ACV with oil, mustard, and other ingredients.
-To make boiled or poached eggs: Add ACV to water to increase its acidity.
-To marinade meat: Combine ACV with other ingredients such as garlic, wine, and spices.
-To replace egg: Add ACV to vegan baking recipes.

WHAT ARE THE HEALTH BENEFITS OF APPLE CIDER VINEGAR?

As if being a useful tool in cooking, cleaning, and self-care wasn't enough, apple cider vinegar offers many health benefits when consumed, especially when it's unfiltered or 'raw'. Raw apple cider vinegar contains additional protein, enzymes, and beneficial bacteria that increase its health benefits.

Here are some of the proven health benefits of apple cider vinegar:

-Lowers blood sugar and improves insulin function, making it very useful for those with diabetes or pre-diabetics.
-Aids in weight loss and reduces belly fat. Consuming ACV with high carb foods increases the feeling of fullness, resulting in less consumption.
-Improves heart health. ACV lowers cholesterol and blood pressure, which reduces the risk of heart disease.
-Protects against cancer. According to some studies, ACV can kill cancer cells and reduce tumors.

In addition to these health benefits, some experts believe that consuming small amounts of apple cider vinegar can aid in digestion. Due to its acidity, ACV helps break down protein and combats harmful bacteria in the stomach. Because of this, Bragg Organic Apple Cider Vinegar has earned a top spot in our bone broth elixir recipes and is a staple ingredient in The Reset Organic Cleanse Program.

You can find Braggs Apple Cider Vinegar in the following products:

-Vegan Mineral Broth Elixir
-Chicken Bone Broth Elixir
-Beef Bone Broth Elixir
-Bison Bone Broth Elixir
-Turkey Bone Broth Elixir

HOW TO INTEGRATE APPLE CIDER VINEGAR INTO YOUR DIET

In addition to eating foods that contain apple cider vinegar, many people choose to take doses of pure apple cider vinegar. To introduce this practice into your wellness regimen, use the following tips:

-Start with small amounts and work up to taking 2 tablespoons per day with meals.
-Protect your teeth by diluting the ACV with water and consuming through a straw.
-Rinse your mouth after consuming.